THIS BOOK

BELONGS TO

....

....

Thank you for Purchasing my book and taking the time to read it from front to back. I am always grateful when a reader chooses my work and I hope you enjoyed it!

With the vast selection available online, I am touched that you chose to be purchasing my work and take valuable time out of your life to read it. My hope is that you feel you made the right decision.

I very much would like to know what you thought of the book. Please take the time to write an honest and informative review on Amazon.com. Your experience and opinions will be of great benefit to me and those readers looking to make an informed choice.

With much thanks.

@COPYRIGHT 2024

Table of Contents

HOW TO DO THE 10-DAY GREEN SMOOTHIE CLEANSE

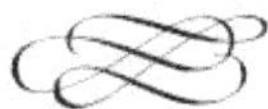

5 DETOX METHODS TO ENHANCE YOUR CLEANSING

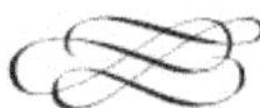

MACA Seed and Avocado Smoothie
Green Salad Smoothie
Natural Energizer Smoothie
Green Herbs Smoothie
Banana, Mint, and Basil Leave Smoothie
Raspberry and Spinach Smoothie
Cabbage, Celery and Pineapple Smoothie
Tropical Refreshing Smoothie
Grape Fruit Smoothie
Easy Green Smoothie
Energizing Green Smoothie
Vanilla Lime Green Smoothie
Rich Fruit Smoothie
Green Fruit Smoothie
Pear and Avocado Smoothie
Bok Choy Smoothie

WHAT IS THE 10-DAY PALEO GREEN SMOOTHIE CLEANSE

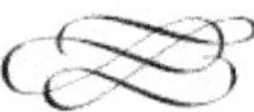

A 10-day green smoothie cleanse is a detoxifying process that ensures weight loss in ten days. In this process, you will consume some delicious green smoothies by blending some finest green vegetables, fruits, and other added ingredients that cleanse your mental and physical health. The 10-day cleanse process will make you lose 10 pounds in ten days without spontaneously exercising at the gym.

This Detox program is designed to kick-start the metabolism to lose weight by burning more fats and calories. Many people often refer it to a fast, which is a misleading concept. Unlike, the starvation the smoothies cleanse gives your digestive system a little break from digesting heavy meals.

Overall body detoxification is the first process to lose weight or to increase the metabolism. And removing the toxins from the body is really hard just by exercising or dieting alone. Therefore, the first step is to cleanse and for that the most effective way is utilizing raw vegetables and fruits.

Now a problem comes how to incorporate the fruits and vegetable daily in the meal. Well, the answer is here in this book. After 10-day cleanse, you will never worry about following any diet plans or measuring calories, as your body mechanism will naturally crave healthy, organic and natural foods.

This handy 10-day cleanse plan will make you go from fat to fit by making your taste buds having a roller coaster ride of flavours. You will get the entire essential nutrient like iron, protein, vitamins, calcium, and phosphorus in the easiest form.

Be a leader and transform your lifestyle by adopting this cleanse program that heals your inner and helps you achieve your weight loss goals.

~

WHY GREEN SMOOTHIES

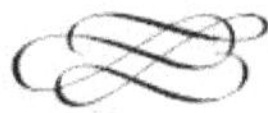

We all drink liquids daily to keep hydrated. But if the water is not providing the energy you needed; then the 10-day smoothie cleanse is surely a gateway to success. And it is a very inexpensive and versatile way to clean the body and flush the toxins from the blood. Many people would think that why green smoothies? Well, why not.

If you want to fulfil the dream of the sexy bikini body, if you want to revitalize the skin, if you want glowing hairs, and need perfect energy to start the day, then the green smoothies cleanse is just for you.

Moreover, green smoothies are rich in fibres, minerals and nutrients that get absorbed much quickly, and easily digested and consumed.

Liquid delivered straight to your cells to start the cleansing process at once. There are many health benefits of green smoothies, few of them

Listed below.

It reduces the signs of aging.
Improve the athletic performance by proving more energy.
Reduce hair loss.
Revitalize the skin.

Improve illness like heart diseases, diabetes, and kidney failure.
Reduce stress and depression.
Reduce anxiety.
Better Sleep.

~

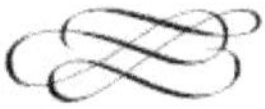

Green smoothie cleanse is a new trend and everyone seems in fashion. Many athletes and celebrities are trying the green smoothie diet for better health and fitness. So indulge yourself in a mouth-watering ten days experience of detoxifying and healing the inner. Get up and feel

More energy
Improved immune system
Better sleep
Improved digestive system
Shiny hairs and glowing skin
Reduced body fat
Reduced inflammation
Reduce hunger pangs
Reduced stress and anxiety

Your biggest do-over is just a few steps away. In the next chapter, you will find ten days green smoothies, prepared from the most organic and fresh ingredients available.

HOW TO DO THE 10-DAY GREEN SMOOTHIE CLEANSE

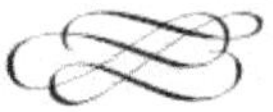

Drink up to 60 ounces of smoothies per day.

Prepare green smoothies enough for the entire day in the morning and pack up to take it with you.

Drink the smoothies as you get hungry or sip 12 to 16 ounces every 4 hours throughout the day.

Try chewing your smoothies as much as you can to avoid bloating and gas.

Chew your smoothies as much as possible, to avoid gas and bloating

You may snack on healthy foods such as crunchy veggies, raw and unsalted nuts and seeds, unsweetened peanut butter, cucumbers, celery and apples throughout the day.

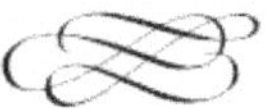

Veggies

All dark leafy green vegetables, asparagus, cauliflower, cabbage, Brussels sprouts, broccoli, carrots, celery, kale, lettuce, spinach, collards, cucumbers, parsley, zucchini

Fruits

All fresh fruits are healthy. However, for weight loss, choose low-sugar fruits such as grapefruits, blueberries, blackberries, cranberries, strawberries, raspberries, passion fruit, limes, lemons.

Milk

Almond milk, coconut milk, hemp milk, goat's milk, oat milk

Nuts and seeds (Raw and unsalted)

Nuts: almonds, cedar nuts, cashews, macadamia, hazelnuts, pecans, peanuts, Brazil nuts, pistachios, walnuts

Seeds: sunflower seeds, pumpkin seeds, hemp seeds, flaxseeds, chia seeds, sesame seeds.

Oils

Extra virgin olive oil, coconut oil, avocado oil, fish oil, flaxseed oil, sesame oil

Sweeteners

Stevia or raw honey

Snacks

Fresh fruits & veggies, lightly salted popcorn, nuts and seeds, organic unsweetened chocolate, almond butter, cashew butter/ peanut butter

Beverages

Spring or distilled water, coconut water, fresh-squeezed juices, green tea, black tea, mint tea/ other herbal teas

Superfood Additions for Smoothies

Aloe Vera, acai berries, avocado, chia seeds, cayenne pepper, goji berries, ginger, flaxseed oil, coconut oil, raw chocolate, fresh wheatgrass juice, sprouts, maca root, or pomegranate juice

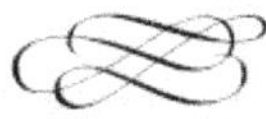

During the challenge, avoid starchy veggies such as beets, carrots, sweet potatoes, and all non-leafy greens.

Processed and refined foods

Refined sugar

Refined carbs such as pastas, breads, donuts, etc.

Animal foods such as meats

Dairy such as milk, cheese, cream, butter, etc.

Dehydrating beverages such as coffee, liquor, beer, sodas, diet sodas, etc.

Fried foods

Your Daily Routine

Start your day off by taking 2 to 3 glasses of water to replenish what you lost overnight.

Follow with one cup of detox tea (herbal teas such as matcha green tea, ginger tea, peppermint tea, chamomile tea, ginseng tea, dandelion tea, etc.),to cleanse your kidneys and liver. You may want to add stevia to your tea to enhance the taste.

Make sure you drink at least 8 glasses of water as well as detox tea per day during the ten-day detox period.

For the first two to four days, you'll fee irritable and hungry. Snack on the healthy foods mentioned earlier to help your body adjust to less and healthy foods. Snacking will help you overcome hunger, but overdoing it will hinder you from losing weight.

You may experience typical detoxification symptoms such as irritability, skin rashes, muscle aches, fatigue, cravings, nausea, pains and headaches.

In case of very strong detox symptoms, follow these guidelines:

Adjust the ratio of vegetables to fruits –begin with 70% fruit to 30% veggies and work your way up to less fruit and more greens over time.

Keep hydrated –drink a lot of water to help ease the detox process.

Ease slowly into the full detox –on the first day, drink a glass of green smoothie for breakfast and have light, healthy meals for both lunch and dinner (salads).By healthy, I mean, avoid dairy, meats, and sugar. On the second day, take green smoothies for both breakfast and lunch and a light healthy meal for dinner. By the third day, you'll be fine to resume with the smoothies all day.

Summary of Your Daily Schedule:

•6:30 AM: Drink 2 to 3 glasses of water

•6:45 AM: Morning Walk

•7 AM: Breakfast Smoothie

•10 AM: Healthy Morning Snack + 2 to 3 glasses of water

•1:30 PM: Lunch Smoothie

•3 PM: Healthy PM Snack + 2 to 3 glasses of water

•4:30 PM: Evening Walk

•6:30 PM: Dinner Smoothie (drink your dinner smoothie at least 2 hours before bedtime)

•8:30 PM: Healthy Bedtime Snack + 2 to 3 glasses of water

BREAKING THE PROGRAM

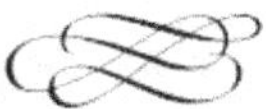

To stay on the right track, avoid going back to eating whole foods right after the ten-day cleanse. Start with salads for at least three days after completing the challenge before introducing whole foods. Continue drinking the green smoothies and check which foods are fine with you. Within the first two days after the challenge, drink a glass of smoothie for breakfast and eat sautéed veggies or salads for lunch and dinner. The objective is to eat light and healthy meals. On the third day after the detox, have a glass of smoothie for breakfast and light meals such as salads and lean healthy meats such as chicken or fish for lunch and dinner. Introduce whole foods on the fourth day but keep them light and healthy.

To maintain long tern weight loss, make it a habit to start your day with a glass of green smoothie for breakfast.

How to Continue Losing Weight after the 10-Day Challenge

Continue losing at least two pounds a week by drinking two green smoothies per day and eating at least one high-protein meal.

HEALTH BENEFITS OF THE 10-DAY GREEN SMOOTHIE WEIGHT LOSS PROGRAM

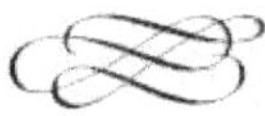

Besides weight loss, our 10-day green smoothie weight loss program reduces the risks for: constipation, bloating, allergies, brain fog, headaches, food cravings, indigestion, yeast infections, sensitivities, chronic pain, and insomnia.

As usual, this program is not designed to place any professional medical treatment for any condition. Consult your physician before embarking on the program.

YOUR DAILY MEAL GUIDE

Keep an eye on the amount of calories you consume for each meal to achieve your weight loss target.

Women (daily allowance 1400kcal)
- Breakfast: 280kcal
- Lunch: 420kcal
- Dinner: 420kcal
- Snacks: 280kcal

Men (daily allowance 1,900kcal)
- Breakfast: 380kcal
- Lunch: 570kcal
- Dinner: 570kcal
- Snacks: 380kcal

If drink more for your breakfast, lunch and dinner smoothie, drop a snack later in the day to stay on track.

~

SHOPPING LIST FOR TEN DAYS

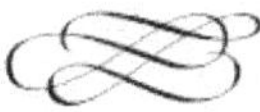

2 ½ cups mango
8 cucumbers
2 sticks of celery
51 ounces spinach
4 cups coconut water
2 cups orange juice
½ tablespoon ginger
2-½ cups pineapple chunks
6 ½ teaspoons of lemon juice
1 cup greens
8 ounces of parsley
2 ounces of mint
4 cups broccoli
8 apples
6 avocados
4-3/4 cups of almond milk
1 lemon
1 cup diced peaches
3 cups water
½ cup green tea
1 cup cilantro
10 ounces kale

¼ cup rolled oats
1 tablespoon of lime juice
1 banana
½ scoop Vega Choc-a-Lot
1 tablespoon flax seeds
4 dates
1 teaspoon vanilla
1 pear

Simply follows these 10 recipes, each for one day and feel the difference yourself.

DAY 1: SPINACH, MANGO, AND COCONUT WATER SMOOTHIE

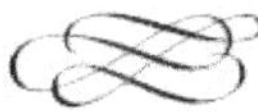

Yield: 4 Servings
Preparation Time: 5 Servings

Ingredients

1 cup fresh spinach
2 cups coconut water, unsweetened
2 cups fresh orange juice
½ cup mango, fresh
½ cup pineapple chunks
½ teaspoon of lemon juice
Ice cubes for chilling

Directions

Place all of your ingredients in a blender.
Blend for 40 seconds.
Pour into serving glasses and enjoy.
Serve chilled.

Nutrition Information per serving

Serving size: 315 g
Calories: 121
Total fat: 0.7g
Cholesterol: 0 mg
Sodium: 134mg
Carb: 27.6g
Protein: 2.2g

DAY 2: THINK GREEN

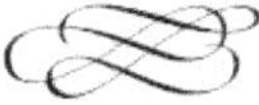

Preparation Time: 5 Minutes
Yield: 2 Servings

Ingredients

2 cups coconut water, cold
1 cup greens, rough chopped
1 ounce of parsley
1 ounce of mint
2 cucumbers, diced
4 small apples, cored and diced
1 cup diced peaches
Ice cubes, for chilling

Directions

Add all the listed ingredients into the blender and pulse for 40 seconds.
Pour into glasses and enjoy.

Nutrition Information per serving

Serving size: 980 g
Calories: 299
Total fat: 1.8g
Cholesterol: 0mg
Sodium: 284mg
Carb: 73.1g
Protein: 6.6g

DAY 3: AVOCADO SMOOTHIE

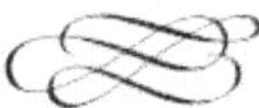

Preparation Time: 5 Minutes
Yield: 6 Servings

Ingredients

1 cup of spinach, fresh
1 cup of almond milk
3 avocados, pits removed
1 ounce of mint
1 cup water
1 cup of ice cubes

Directions

Pour almond milk into the blender.
Chop the avocados and add to the blender.
Then add other listed ingredients.
Pulse for 30 seconds or until smooth.
Transfer the smoothie into ice-filled glasses and enjoy.

Nutrition Information per serving

Serving size: 190g
Calories: 300

Total fat: 29.2g
Cholesterol: 0mg
Sodium: 19mg
Carb: 11.4g
Protein: 3.1g

~

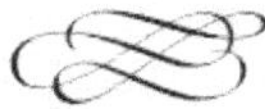

Preparation Time: 5 Minutes
Yield: 6 Servings

Ingredients

4 apples, peeled and cubed
2 cups of celery, washed
2 cucumbers, washed
2 avocados, pitted
1 cup spinach, washed
4 cups water

Directions

Wash and peel the apples.
Wash all other vegetables and pit the avocados.
Then, place all the listed ingredients in a blender
Pulse it for a few minutes.
Then serve in ice-filled glasses and enjoy.

Nutrition Information per serving

Serving size: 367g

Calories: 221
Total fat: 13.5g
Cholesterol: 0mg
Sodium: 39mg
Carb: 27.3g
Protein: 2.6g

DAY 5: GO GREEN SMOOTHIE

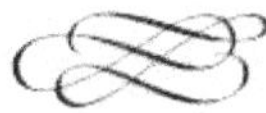

Preparation Time: 5 Minutes
Yield: 2 Servings

Ingredients

4 cups broccoli
1 ounce of parsley, washed
1 ounce of spinach, washed
1 lemon, peeled and cut into wedges
Salt, pinch
1 cup water
Ice cubes, for chilling
Directions

Blend all the listed ingredients in a blender, stir and pour into ice-filled glasses.
Enjoy the perfect sip of mouth-watering smoothie.

Nutrition Information per serving

Serving size: 253g
Calories: 83
Total fat: 0.9g

Cholesterol: 0 mg\
Sodium: 157mg\
Carb: 17g\
Protein: 6.4g

~

DAY 6: DETOX SMOOTHIE

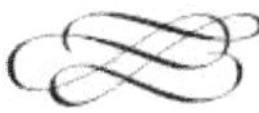

Preparation Time: 3 Minutes
Yield: 4 Servings

Ingredients

½ cup green tea, chilled
1 cup cilantro
1 cup organic kale
2 cups cucumber
1 cup pineapple
1-ounce lemon juice
½ tablespoon fresh ginger
1 avocado, pitted
1 cup water

Preparation

Place ingredients in a blender and pulse until smooth.
Serve into glasses and enjoy.

Nutrition Information per serving

Serving size: 322g

Calories: 144
Total fat: 10g
Cholesterol: 0 mg
Sodium: 15mg
Carb: 14.5g
Protein: 2.2g

DAY 7: A GREEN START

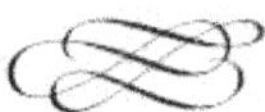

Preparation Time: 5 Minutes
Yield: 3 Servings

Ingredients

½ banana, peeled
1 cup almond milk
2 ounces spinach
¼ cup rolled oats, raw
½ scoop Vega Choc-a-Lot
1 tablespoon flax seed
Ice cubes for chilling

Topping

Granola

Directions

Place ingredients in a blender and puree until smooth.
Serve into glasses with a garnish of granola.

Nutrition Information per serving

Serving size: 132g

Calories: 259
Total fat: 20.4g
Cholesterol: 0mg
Sodium: 52mg
Carb: 15.7g
Protein: 6.4g

DAY 8: SHAMROCK SMOOTHIE

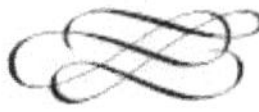

Preparation Time: 2 Minutes
Yield: 6 Servings

Ingredients

3 cups almond milk, unsweetened
1 cup spinach
½ cup mint
¼ cup banana, peeled
4 dates, pitted
1 teaspoon vanilla

Directions

Blend all listed ingredients in a blender until smooth.
Pour into glasses and enjoy.

Nutrition Information per serving

Serving size: 145g
Calories: 304
Total fat: 28g
Cholesterol: 0 mg

Sodium: 24mg
Carb: 13.1g
Protein: 3.4g

DAY 9: HAPPY GREEN MONSTER

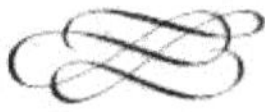

Preparation Time: 5 Minutes
   Yield: 2-3 Servings

Ingredients

1 cup almond milk
1 pear, peeled and cored
2 ounces kale
Ice cubes, for chilling

Directions

Blend all listed ingredients in a blender until smooth.
Enjoy.

Nutrition Information per serving

Serving size: 145 g
Calories: 220
Total fat: 19.1g
Cholesterol: 0 mg
Sodium: 21mg
Carb: 13.5g

Protein: 2.6 g

DAY 10: LUCK GREEN SMOOTHIE

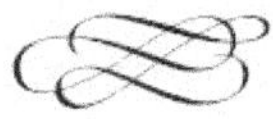

Preparation Time: 5 Minutes
Yield: 2 Servings

Ingredients

2 cups fresh spinach
2 cups water
207 g or 2 cups mango, frozen
1 cup pineapple

Instructions

Toss all ingredients in a blender.
Add water and blend together.
Pour into serving glasses and enjoy.

Nutrition Information per serving

Serving size: 557 g
Calories: 193
Total fat: 0.8g
Cholesterol: 0 mg
Sodium: 36mg

Carb: 47.1g
Protein: 2.3g

∽

PERSONAL TIPS FOR SUCCESS

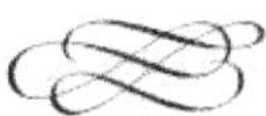

Listed below are some personal tips that make your weight loss process more effective.

Tip 1: While preparing the smoothies, try using water or coconut water. Use almond milk because it helps you lose weight and gives the smoothie a creamy texture. You can also use Greek yogurt as it makes the smoothie more tempting. Try adding extra nutrients by including hemp seed, Chia seeds or flax seed. The fats from nuts are good and it doesn't make you obese. The plant-based fat has always affected positive on the body and initiates weight loss.

Tip 2: Try keeping the fat content low by adding more vegetable and fruits and fewer nuts and seeds. The excess fat may cause gas and bloat.

Tip 3: Always use artificial zero-calorie sweeter in your smoothies if needed. Instead of artificial stuff, try adding sweet fruits like bananas or mangoes. These fruits will sweeten the smoothie and you will not need any artificial stuff.

Tip 4: Skip the agave nectar, honey or maple syrup as much as you can. All these are concentrated sugar leads to weight gains. Try dates, bananas or mangoes instead.

Tip 5: Use protein powders that boost the protein content. It helps you feel full for a longer time.

Tip 6: Make a rich glass of smoothie that serves as a meal replacement.

Tip 7: Stick with organic, fresh, whole fruits, vegetables, and leafy greens. Avoid canned fruit as much as possible as the syrup in them leads to excess sugar.

Tip 8: "Go Green" is the symbol you should adopt for better health and fitness.

HOW TO CONTINUE TO LOSE WEIGHT AFTER THE CLEANSE

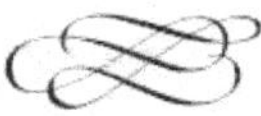

A lot of people adopt smoothie cleanse to lose weight, but then stop indulging themselves to it afterward. So it is being advised to first not entirely stick to the diet plan if you find it hard afterward.

Here are a few tips.

•Try replacing one of your meals with smoothie glass. Because when you fill your body with tons of nutrients, then you can easily fight hunger pangs.

•Avoid junk food items during and after smoothie cleanse.

•Along with smoothie diet, it is recommended to eat a low fat and a reasonable meal to make the weight loss process more effective.

•It's recommended to eat on time.

•Avoid drinking water during the meal.

•Avoid intake of red meat, pork, and beef.

•Choose healthy oil options for cooking.

•Half of your serving plate should fill with fruits and vegetables.

•Try not to skip a meal.

•Check the food labels before buying any food item at grocery stores.

•Go for organic food choices.

•Say no to sodas, and other beverages available in the market.

•Drink plenty of water throughout the day.

5 DETOX METHODS TO ENHANCE YOUR CLEANSING

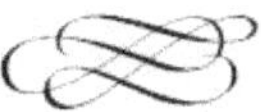

Despite being on smoothies cleanse plan, numerous ways are available to detoxify the body, few have listed below.

Start Day by Drinking Water

Start your day with a glass of water. The water keeps you hydrated. Adding a few drops of lemon keep you hydrated and also cleanses the toxins out of the body.

Combat Environmental Pollution

There is a lot of air pollution around you, which leads to certain allergies like puffy eyes, red nose, and sneezing. Clear your nasal passage daily before going to bed.

Sweat it out

If you are on a cleanse program, then try spending ten minutes in a sauna three days a week. Try to drink water and keep checking with your doctor.

Eat clean

Almost everything you buy in the tins packs is processed, so try to keep away from all processed and packed food items. Go for organic and fresh food items. Sure, right food will do right to your body.

Exercise regularly

The exercise regulates the blood circulation and doing so enhance the digestive system. Exercise reduces tension, and people who exercising regularly had far less toxic in their bodies. Exercise help burns calories and keeps you in shape.

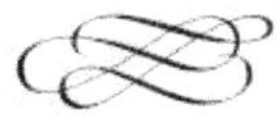

PINEAPPLE, SPINACH AND STRAWBERRY SMOOTHIE

Preparation Time: 5 Minutes
    Yield: 4 Servings

Ingredients

1 cup low-fat vanilla yogurt
1 cup water
1 cup pineapple chunks
1 cup strawberries
1 cup spinach, lightly packed
Ice cubes for chilling

Directions

Add all the listed ingredients in the blender and pulse until smooth.

Pour into the tall serving glasses.

Enjoy.

Nutrition Information per serving

Serving size: 205g
Calories: 77
Total fat: 0.9g
Cholesterol: 4 mg
Sodium: 51mg
Carb: 12.8g
Protein: 4.2g

FALL GREEN SMOOTHIE

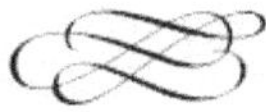

Preparation Time: 5 Minutes
  Yield: 4 Servings

Ingredients

2 cups kale
2 cups pear, peeled
1 cup green grapes
2 tablespoons of cashew
1 cup almond milk

Directions

Remove the seeds of pears.
Blend kale, pears, grapes, cashew and almond milk in a blender.
Once a smooth texture obtained, pour into glasses.
Serve and enjoy.

Nutrition Information per serving

Serving size: 201 g
Calories: 241
Total fat: 16.5g
Cholesterol: 0mg

Sodium: 26 mg
Carb: 24.4 g
Protein: 3.5g

SPINACH AND ALMOND MILK SMOOTHIE

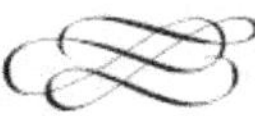

Preparation Time: 10 Minutes
Yield: 4 Servings

Ingredients

2 tablespoons almond butter, unsalted
1 cup of spinach, fresh
1 cup of almond milk
1 cup pineapple, chunks
1 teaspoon of Chia seed
1 cup of ice cubes

Directions

Combine all the listed ingredients in a blender and pulse until smooth.
Pour into ice-filled glasses.
Enjoy.

Nutrition Information per serving

Serving size: 117g
Calories: 213
Total fat: 19.1g

Cholesterol: 0 mg
Sodium: 15mg
Carb: 10.7g
Protein: 3.6 g

MINT BLAST

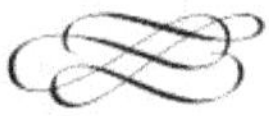

Preparation Time: 5 Minutes
Yield: 1 Serving

Ingredients

2 kiwis, peeled
1 ounce of mint, fresh
1 cucumber
1 cup of water, filtered

Directions

Place the kiwis, mint, and cucumber in a blender.
Pour in the water.
Pulse the blender until smooth.
Pour into ice-filled glasses and enjoy.
Serve Immediately.

Nutrition Information per serving

Serving size: 718g
Calories: 150
Total fat: 1.3g
Cholesterol: 0mg

Sodium: 26mg
Carb: 35g
Protein: 4.6g

GRAPE BASIL SMOOTHIE

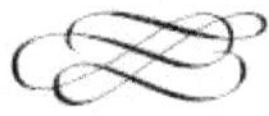

Preparation Time: 5 Minutes
Yield: 4 Servings

Ingredients

2 cups green grapes
½ inch chunk of ginger, peeled and chopped
1-ounce of basil, fresh
½ cup of sunflower seeds
1 lime, juiced
1 cup water, filtered

Directions

Transfer all the listed ingredients in the blender.
Pulse it until a smooth texture is formed.
Serve into ice-filled glasses and enjoy.

Nutrition Information per serving

Serving size: 135g
Calories: 73
Total fat: 3.2g
Cholesterol: 0mg

Sodium: 4mg
Carb: 11.3g
Protein: 1.9g

APPLE CUCUMBER SMOOTHIE

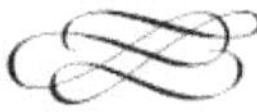

Preparation Time: 5 Minutes
Yield: 4 Servings

Ingredients

1cup green apples, cubes
½-inch ginger
1 cup of cucumber, peeled and chopped
1 tablespoon of mint leaves
1 cup of celery sticks
6 Ice cubes, for chilling
½ cup water

Directions

Wash all the vegetables and fruits.
Peel the apples and remove seeds.
Peel the cucumber and finely chop.
Place cucumber, apples, ginger, honey, mint, and celery in a blender.
Add ice cubes and water.
Pulse mixture for 40 seconds.

Once the desired consistency obtained, pour into ice-filled serving glasses and enjoy.

Nutrition Information per serving

Serving size: 110g
Calories: 23
Total fat: 0.1g
Cholesterol: 0 mg
Sodium: 15mg
Carb: 5.7g
Protein: 0.3g

GRANNY SMITH SMOOTHIE

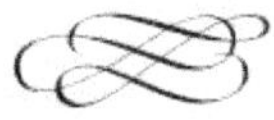

Preparation Time: 5 Minutes
Yield: 4 Servings

Ingredients
2 cups spinach, washed
2 granny smith apples, peeled and cored
1 cup water

Directions
Combine spinach, apples, and water in a blender.
Pulse until desired consistency obtained.
Serve into ice-filled glasses and enjoy.

Nutrition Information per serving
Serving size: 331g
Calories: 105
Total fat: 0.5g
Cholesterol: 0 mg
Sodium: 29mg
Carb: 26.2g
Protein: 1.4g

MIX VEGETABLES SMOOTHIE

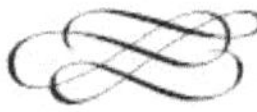

Preparation Time: 5 Minutes
Yield: 4 Servings

Ingredients

1 cup spinach
2 cucumbers
1 cup water
1 cup kale
Ice cubes, for chilling

Direction

Combine all the listed ingredients in the blender and pulse until smooth.
Pour into tall smoothie glasses and enjoy.

Nutrition Information per serving

Serving size: 234g
Calories: 33
Total fat: 0.2g
Cholesterol: 0mg

Sodium: 18mg
Carb: 7.5 g
Protein: 1.7g

AVOCADO COCONUT SMOOTHIE

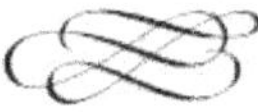

Preparation Time: 5 Minutes
Yield: 2 Servings

Ingredients

2 avocados, pitted
1 cup milk
1-ounce coconut flakes

Directions

Wash and pit the avocados.
Place the avocados along with coconut flakes, and milk in the blender.
Pulse for 40 seconds or until smooth.
Pour into serving glasses and enjoy.

Nutrition Information per serving

Serving size: 169 g
Calories: 261
Total fat: 23.2 g
Cholesterol: 5mg

Sodium: 36 mg
Carb: 12.7g
Protein: 4.2g

KALE CHERRY SMOOTHIE

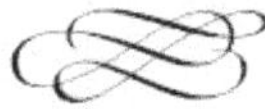

Preparation Time: 5 Minutes
Yield: 4 Servings

Ingredients

1 cup frozen cherries
2 cups kale stems removed
2 cups water
2 tablespoons of hemp seeds
1 cup ice cubes, for chilling

Directions

Add all the listed ingredients into a blender and blend on high for about 30 seconds or until you reach a smooth and creamy consistency.

Pour into serving glasses and enjoy.

Nutrition Information per serving

Serving size: 254g
Calories: 55
Total fat: 1.9g
Cholesterol: 0 mg

Sodium: 20mg
Carb: 8g
Protein: 2.6 g

SUMMER SMOOTHIE

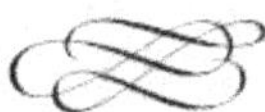

Preparation Time: 5 Minutes
Yield: 1 Serving

Ingredients

2 cups cucumbers, washed
Pinch of salt
Pinch of black pepper
1 tablespoon of lemon juice
½ cup water

Directions

Wash and peel the cucumber.
Add cucumber, salt, pepper and lemon juice in a blender.
Pour water into the blender.
Blend mixture on high speed for about 30 seconds or until you reach a smooth and creamy consistency.
Pour into serving glasses and enjoy.

Nutrition Information per serving

Serving size: 342g
Calories: 35

Total fat: 0.3g
Cholesterol: 0 mg
Sodium: 166mg
Carb: 7.9g
Protein: 1.5 g

PINEAPPLE AND APPLE SMOOTHIE

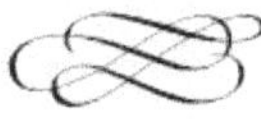

Preparation Time: 5 Minutes
   Yield: 2 Servings

Ingredients

2 green apples, seeds removed
2 cups pineapples, cut and cubed
1 lemon, peeled
½ cup coconut water
Directions

Wash apples and peel the skin.
Remove the seeds of the apple.
Blend all the listed ingredients in a blender.
Once the smoothie is ready, pour into tall glasses and enjoy.

Nutrition Information per serving

Serving size: 415g
Calories: 190
Total fat: 0.7g
Cholesterol: 0 mg
Sodium: 75 mg

Carb: 49.3g
Protein: 1.9g

KALE AND ORANGE SMOOTHIE

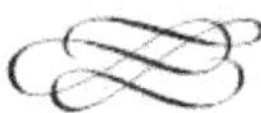

Preparation Time: 5 Minutes
Yield: 6 Servings

Ingredients

4 cups kale, washed
4 oranges, peeled and deseeded
1 cup of ice cubes
1 cup water
½ cup broccoli
Directions

Blend the kale, oranges, and broccoli in a blender.
Pour the water into the blender.
Pulse it for a few seconds.
Pour into the ice-filled glasses.
Serve and enjoy.

Nutrition Information per serving

Serving size: 245g
Calories: 8
Total fat: 0.2g

Cholesterol: 0 mg
Sodium: 24mg
Carb: 19.6g
Protein: 2.7g

CLASSIC SMOOTHIE

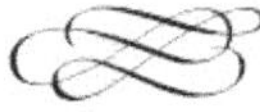

Preparation Time: 5 Minutes
   Yield: 4 Servings

Ingredients

2 cups spinach
1 cup almond milk
2 tablespoons of coconut flakes
3-4 cups pineapple chunks

Directions

Blend spinach, Almond milk, and coconut flakes and pineapples
in a blender.
Blend again.
Pour into the ice-filled glasses.
Serve and enjoy.

Nutrition Information per serving

Serving size: 201 g
Calories: 212
Total fat: 15.4g

Cholesterol: 0 mg
Sodium: 23mg
Carb: 20.5g
Protein: 2.6g

SPINACH ORANGE SMOOTHIE

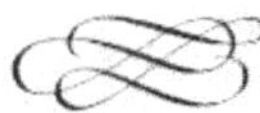

Preparation Time: 2 Minutes
Yield: 2 Servings

Ingredients

2 oranges, peeled
1 banana, peeled
2 cups organic spinach
1 cup coconut water, adjusted as desired
Ice cubes, for chilling

Directions

Add all ingredients to a blender with a few ice cubes and blend on high for 10 seconds.
Add more coconut water if desired.
Pour into glasses and enjoy.

Nutrition Information per serving

Serving size: 393g
Calories: 169
Total fat: 0.8g
Cholesterol: 0 mg

Sodium: 150mg
Carb: 40.6g
Protein: 4.1g

FRUIT MIX DRINK

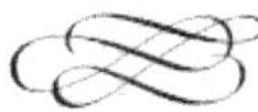

Preparation Time: 5 Minutes
Yield: 3 Servings

Ingredients

2 cups organic fresh apple juice
2 cups of grapes
2 kiwis
Ice cubes, for chilling

Directions

First, you need to wash, and chop the apples and then pass it through the juicer.
Now pour apple juice, kiwis and grapes in a blender and pulse.
Serve in ice-filled glasses and enjoy.

Nutrition Information per serving

Serving size: 277g
Calories: 150
Total fat: 0.7g

Cholesterol: 0mg
Sodium: 8mg
Carb: 37.5g
Protein: 1.1 g

GINGER AND PEAR SMOOTHIE

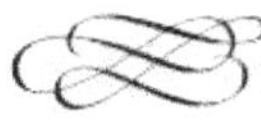

Preparation Time: 5 Minutes
   Yield: 2 Servings

Ingredients

2 large ripe pears
1 ripe banana, peeled
2 cups kale
1 small piece of ginger, peeled
16 ounces kombucha, citrus flavour
2 cups water

Directions

Wash and remove the seeds of pears.
Blend all the listed ingredients in the blender and pulse.
Pour into serving glasses and enjoy.

Nutrition Information per serving

Serving size: 325g
Calories: 116
Total fat: 0.4g
Cholesterol: 0mg

Sodium: 16mg
Carb: 29g
Protein: 1.4g

KALE AND ALMOND MILK SMOOTHIE

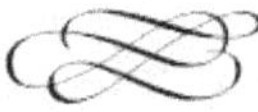

Preparation Time: 5 Minutes
Yield: 2 Servings

Ingredients

2 cups kale
2 tablespoons of cashew
1 cup almond milk

Directions

Blend all listed ingredients in a blender until smooth.
Pour into ice-filled serving glasses.
Enjoy.

Nutrition Information per serving

Serving size: 196
Calories: 358
Total fat: 0g
Cholesterol: 0 mg
Sodium: 48mg
Carb: 16g
Protein: 6.1g

MANGO AND SPINACH SMOOTHIE

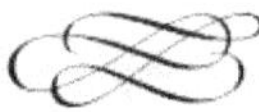

Preparation Time: 5 Minutes
Yield: 2 Servings

Ingredients

1 cup spinach leaves, fresh washed
1 cup frozen mango, cubes
1 cup almond milk
½ cup orange juice
½ cup ice cubes
2 tablespoons of honey

Directions

Blend all listed ingredients in a blender until smooth.
Pour into ice-filled serving glasses.
Enjoy.

Nutrition Information per serving

Serving size: 381g
Calories: 444
Total fat: 29g
Cholesterol: 0mg

Sodium: 35 mg
Carb: 48g
Protein: 4.2g

HEALTHY SMOOTHIE

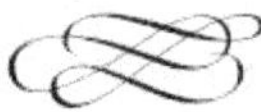

Preparation Time: 5 Minutes
Yield: 2 Servings

Ingredients

1 cup unsweetened almond milk
1/3 cup non-fat plain yogurt
1 cup baby spinach
½ cup frozen pineapple chunks
1 tablespoon chia seeds

Directions

Blend all listed ingredients in the blender until smooth.
Pour into ice-filled serving glasses.
Enjoy.

Nutrition Information per serving

Serving size: 292g
Calories: 183
Total fat: 7.2g
Cholesterol: 2 mg

Sodium: 132mg
Carb: 23g
Protein: 6.7 g

APPLE AND PECAN SMOOTHIE

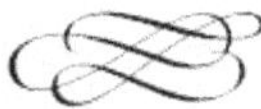

Yield: 2 Servings
Preparation Time: 3 Minutes

Ingredients

2 green apples
2 avocados, pitted
2 pieces of pecans, unsalted
2 tablespoons of cashews
1 cup of water
4 ice cubes, for chilling
1/3 teaspoon of nutmeg

Directions

Blend all the listed ingredients in a blender for about 40 seconds.
Serve into ice-filled tall glasses and enjoy.
Best served chilled.

Nutrition Information per serving

Serving size: 256g
Calories: 283

Total fat: 22.3g
Cholesterol: 0mg
Sodium: 9 mg
Carb: 22.8g
Protein: 2.9g

MACA SEED AND AVOCADO SMOOTHIE

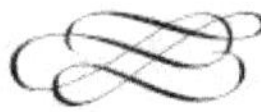

Yield: 4 Servings
Preparation Time: 5 Minutes

Ingredients

2 avocados, pitted
1 cup blueberries
1 cup of water
2 teaspoons of MACA powder
Ice cubes, as needed

Directions

Blend all the listed ingredients in a blender for 30 seconds.
Pour into the smoothie glasses and enjoy.
Best served chilled.

Nutrition Information per serving

Serving size: 198 g
Calories: 232
Total fat: 19.8g
Cholesterol: 0mg
Sodium: 8mg

Carb: 13.9g
Protein: 2.4g

GREEN SALAD SMOOTHIE

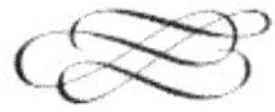

Yield: 2 Servings
Preparation Time: 4 Minutes

Ingredients

1 Habanero pepper, seeds removed
2 cucumbers
2 cups green cabbage
1 tablespoon of lemon juice, fresh and juiced
1 ounce of parsley, fresh and roughly torn
2 mint leaves
½ ounce of kale, de-stemmed
1 cup water, filtered
5 to 6 ice cubes

Directions

Wash the vegetables before making a smoothie.
Pulse all the listed ingredients together in a blender.
Pour into serving glasses and enjoy this refreshing drink.

Nutrition Information per serving

Serving size: 272g
Calories: 42
Total fat: 0.4g
Cholesterol: 0mg
Sodium: 19 mg
Carb: 9.5g
Protein: 2.0g

NATURAL ENERGIZER SMOOTHIE

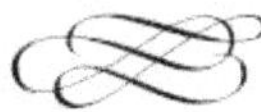

Preparation Time: 5 Minutes
Yield: 4 Servings
Ingredients
1 cup pineapple, chunks
2 cups spinach
1 cucumber
1 cup ice cubes
1 cup of celery, chopped
1 cup fennel, chunk
Pinch of salt

Directions

Wash the vegetables and fruits well before making a smoothie.
Place all the listed ingredients in a blender and pulse for 30 seconds.
Once the smoothie is prepared, pour into tall serving glasses and enjoy.

Nutrition Information per serving

Serving size: 238g
Calories: 46

Total fat: 0.3g
Cholesterol: 0mg
Sodium: 86mg
Carb: 11g
Protein: 1.6g

GREEN HERBS SMOOTHIE

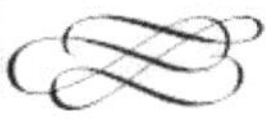

Yield: 2-3servings
Preparation Time: 5 Minute

Ingredients

1 ounce of mint, fresh
1 ounce of basil
1 ounce of parsley
1 cup of water, filtered
2 cups pineapple juice
Ice cubes for chilling

Directions

Place all of your ingredients into a blender.
Blend for 50 seconds.
Pour into tall glasses and serve.
Enjoy.

Nutrition Information per serving

Serving size: 411g
Calories: 147
Total fat: 0.6 g

Cholesterol: 0 mg
Sodium: 21 mg
Carb: 34.6 g
Protein: 2.2g

BANANA, MINT, AND BASIL LEAVE SMOOTHIE

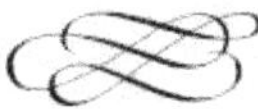

Preparation Time: 5 Minutes
Yield: 2 Servings

Ingredients

1 banana, peeled
2 ounces of basil leaves, fresh
2 cups water
4 ounces of mint leaves

Directions

Pour all the listed ingredients in the blender and pulse for 20 seconds.
Serve into glasses and enjoy.
Best served chilled.

Nutrition Information per serving

Serving size: 381g
Calories: 84
Total fat: 0.8g
Cholesterol: 8 mg

Sodium: 26mg
Carb: 19 g
Protein: 3.4

RASPBERRY AND SPINACH SMOOTHIE

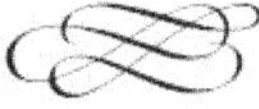

Preparation Time: 5 Minutes
   Yield: 2 Servings

Ingredients

½ cup raw milk, unsweetened
1 cup of yogurt, plain
1 cup raspberries, frozen
2 cups spinach
1 cup kale
1 cup crushed ice

Directions

Blend the entire listed ingredients in a blender and pulse until smooth.
Pour into the ice-filled glasses and serve.

Nutrition Information per serving

Serving size: 309g
Calories: 173
Total fat: 3.3g
Cholesterol: 12 mg

Sodium: 153 mg
Carb: 23g
Protein: 11g

CABBAGE, CELERY AND PINEAPPLE SMOOTHIE

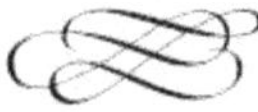

Yield: 2 Servings
Preparation Time: 5 Minutes

Ingredients

2 cups pineapple chunks, frozen
1 cup cabbage, frozen
1 cup celery
1 cup crushed ice

Directions

Blend the entire listed ingredients in a blender and pulse until smooth.
Pour into the ice-filled glasses and serve.

Nutrition Information per serving

Serving size: 251g
Calories: 99
Total fat: 0.3 g
Cholesterol: 0 mg
Sodium: 49mg
Carb: 25.3g

Protein: 1.7g

Peppermint and Celery Smoothie

Preparation Time: 5 Minutes
Yield: 1-2 Servings

Ingredients

2 tablespoons of lemon juice
1 ounce of celery, washed and chopped
1 cup of peppermint leaves, washed
1 cup water

Directions

Blend all the listed ingredients in the blender.
Pulse it for 30 seconds.
Serve into a tall ice-filled glass and enjoy.
Best served chilled.

Nutrition Information per serving

Serving size: 194g
Calories: 26
Total fat: 0.5 g
Cholesterol: 0mg
Sodium: 32mg
Carb: 4.6g
Protein: 1.7g

TROPICAL REFRESHING SMOOTHIE

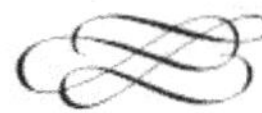

Yield: 1 Serving
Preparation Time: 5 Minutes

Ingredients
1 cup coconut water, unsweetened
1 cup pineapple chunks, frozen
1/3 avocado, pitted
Ice cubes for chilling

Directions
Blend all listed ingredients in a blender until smooth.
Pour into ice-filled serving glasses.
Enjoy.

Nutrition Information per serving
Serving size: 118g
Calories: 66
Total fat: 0.8
Cholesterol: 0mg
Sodium: 65mg
Carb: 9.1g
Protein: 1 g

GRAPE FRUIT SMOOTHIE

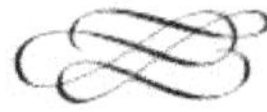

Preparation Time: 5 Minutes
Yield: 4 Servings

Ingredients

2 grapefruits, peeled, seeds removed
2 large sweet apple, cored and skin removed
2 cups spinach, frozen
2 large ripe bananas, sliced and frozen
2-3 ice cubes
2 cups orange juice

Directions

Blend all listed ingredients in a blender until smooth.
Pour into ice-filled serving glasses.
Enjoy.

Nutrition Information per serving

Serving size: 383g
Calories: 198
Total fat: 0.8g
Cholesterol: 0 mg

Sodium: 15 mg
Carb: 4.9g
Protein: 2.7g

EASY GREEN SMOOTHIE

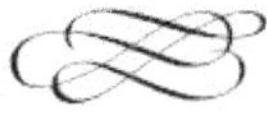

Preparation Time: 5 Minutes
Yield: 4 Servings

Ingredients

2 large green apples, cored and skin removed
2 cups of mango slices, frozen
2 large ripe bananas, sliced and frozen
2-3 ice cubes
4 cups kale
1 cup water

Directions

Blend all listed ingredients in a blender until smooth.
Pour into ice-filled serving glasses.
Enjoy.

Nutrition Information per serving

Serving size: 350g
Calories: 220
Total fat: 0.7g

Cholesterol: 0 mg
Sodium: 33mg
Carb: 55g
Protein: 3.6g

ENERGIZING GREEN SMOOTHIE

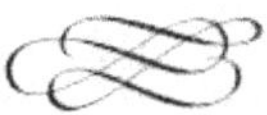

Preparation Time: 5 Minutes
Yield: 6 Servings

Ingredients

1 banana, peeled
1 cup kale
2 cups almond milk
2 tablespoons of Chia seeds
2 tablespoons of shredded coconut
1 tablespoon of almond butter
1 scoop of wheatgrass powder

Directions

Add all the listed ingredients into a high-powered blender.
Blend on high for one minute.
Pour into a tall serving glass and enjoy.

Nutrition Information per serving

Serving size: 150g
Calories: 288
Total fat: 24g

Cholesterol: 0 mg
Sodium: 18 mg
Carb: 15g
Protein: 5.4g

VANILLA LIME GREEN SMOOTHIE

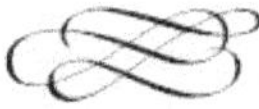

Preparation Time: 5 Minutes
Yield: 2 Servings

Ingredients

1 cup vanilla yogurt
1 cup spinach leaves
1 tablespoon fresh lime juice
½ teaspoon vanilla extract
½ cup milk
2 tablespoons of honey
Ice cubes for chilling

Directions

Place all ingredients except the ice in a blender and puree until smooth.
Serve into ice-filled glasses and enjoy.

Nutrition Information per serving

Serving size: 243g
Calories: 193
Total fat: 2.8g

Cholesterol: 12 mg
Sodium: 128 mg
Carb: 31g
Protein: 9.6 g

RICH FRUIT SMOOTHIE

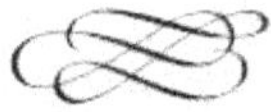

Preparation Time: 5 Minutes
Yield: 4 Servings

Ingredients

2 cups avocados, pitted
1 cup pears, peeled and chopped
2 cups water
2 green apples, peeled
2 cups green grapes
Ice cubes, for chilling

Directions

Wash all the vegetables.
Peel the pears and apples and remove the seeds.
Blend grapes, avocados, pears, apples, and water in a blender.
Blend it until smooth.
Pour into ice-filled serving glasses and enjoy.

Nutrition Information per serving

Serving size: 369g

Calories: 240
Total fat: 14.6g
Cholesterol: 0 mg
Sodium: 10mg
Carb: 32g
Protein: 2.1g

GREEN FRUIT SMOOTHIE

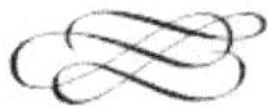

Preparation Time: 5 Minutes
Yield: 2 Servings

Ingredients

2 cups Swiss chard
2 cups pears, peeled and chopped
2 green apples, peeled and deseeded
Ice cubes, for chilling
2 cups water

Directions

Wash all the fruits and vegetable.
Peel the pears and apples and remove the seeds.
Blend apples, grapes, pear, Swiss chard and water in a blender.
Blend mixture until smooth.
Pour into ice-filled serving glasses and enjoy.

Nutrition Information per serving

Serving size: 616g
Calories: 195

Total fat: 0g
Cholesterol: 0mg
Sodium: 88mg
Carb: 51g
Protein: 1.7g

PEAR AND AVOCADO SMOOTHIE

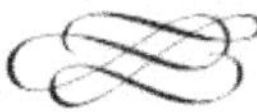

Preparation Time: 5 Minutes
Yield: 4 Servings

Ingredients

2 cups avocados
1 cup pears
2 cups coconut water
2 cups pineapple
Ice cubes, for chilling

Directions

Blend avocados, pears and coconut water in a blender.
Then add the pineapples.
Blend until smooth.
Pour into ice-filled serving glasses and enjoy.

Nutrition Information per serving

Serving size: 316g
Calories: 236
Total fat: 14.6g

Cholesterol: 0mg
Sodium: 132 mg
Carb: 27.7g
Protein: 3g

BOK CHOY SMOOTHIE

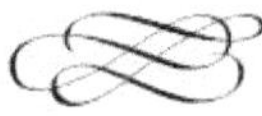

Preparation Time: 5 Minutes
  Yield: 2 Servings

Ingredients

2 cups fresh spinach
2 cups bok Choy
2 cups water
3 cups pear, frozen
1 cup pineapple
Ice cubes, for chilling

Directions

Toss a spinach, water, and bok Choy in a blender.
Pulse it for a while.
Then add remaining ingredients and blend again for 30 seconds.
Pour into ice-filled serving glasses and enjoy.

Nutrition Information per serving

Serving size: 661 g
Calories: 197
Total fat: 0.7g

Cholesterol: 0 mg
Sodium: 80 mg
Carb: 50.2 g
Protein: 3.2g

CONCLUSION

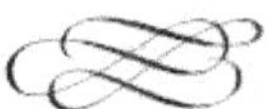

Losing weight is so easy when it comes to 10-day cleanse program. This book surely provides all the essential information and recipes to kick-start the process. So achieve the dream of sexy bikini body by sipping your way through one recipe each day for ten days.

Thank you again for downloading this book!

I hope this book was able to help you to lose your weight, stay healthy and learn about awesome health benefits .The next step is to take action.

Again above is a guideline for you to help getting started? Feel free to change the diets according to your desires. If you follow the tips and try the recipes I shared with you, you will definitely see better and a healthier you.

Again thank you for downloading this book. Spread the good news and enjoy the Awesome Life style today!

Finally, if you've received value from this book, please take the time to share your thoughts and post a review on Amazon. It'd be greatly appreciated!